Doodle Art Sketchbook: Mindful and Calming

Published in the United States of America

978-1-60808-309-1 (p)
978-1-60808-310-7 (e)

Book and cover design by Robin Krauss,
www.bookformatters.com

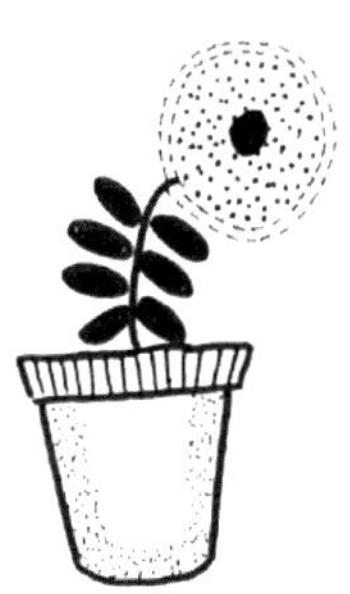

Doodling is thinking in disguise.

— Sunni Brown

Repetition is key because the more you do it the better you feel.

— Melissa Lloyd

Simple, quick, accessible "acts of art" can enhance your life.

— Susan Magsamen and Ivy Ross

Just for You

This book is designed for easy use, with smaller pages and brief prompts.

Tuck it in your pocket, purse, or backpack. When you're feeling bored, anxious, stressed, down, or another emotion, take it out and doodle.

The *Doodle Art Sketchbook* is your buddy, close at hand and with you as you make your way through the day.

This book belongs to

____

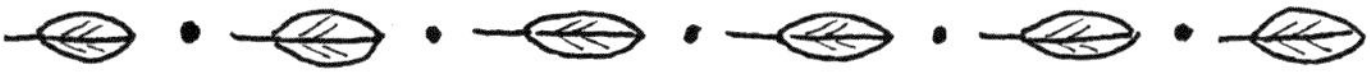

Using This Sketchbook

To sketch, use a pencil, ballpoint pen, colored pencils, or felt-tip marker. The pages are purposely printed on one side so you can sketch on both sides. The *Doodle Art Sketchbook* has many pluses.

- Handy, take-along size.
- Doodle anywhere, anytime.
- Start on any page.
- Set your own pace.
- Packed with info, patterns, and techniques.

Best of all, every doodle is an expression of you.

What is Mindfulness?

The Mindful website, www.mindful.org, defines it this way:

The practice of being fully present and aware of your current experience—without overreacting or getting lost in thought.

The best thing about mindfulness is that it can always be increased. Although you're already mindful, your mindfulness may have lagged lately. Make mindfulness a priority again.

Doodle a lightbulb here for mindfulness.

What is Creativity?

Author Diana Vinther says, "Creativity is a seed, an inborn and imperishable one, which can spread in manifold ways and grow into extraordinary things like the tree inside an acorn . . ."

Just as a tree is inside an acorn, creativity is inside you. Let it out and let it grow.

Doodle an acorn here.

What is Doodling?

Doodling is conscious or subconscious drawing, or a combination of both. When you doodle, you're not sure how it's going to turn out. In case you're wondering, all doodles are abstract, some more than others.

Because the heart shape is used often in doodling, I define it as a melding of ordinary doodling, comic techniques, and folk art.

Doodle here and include a heart.

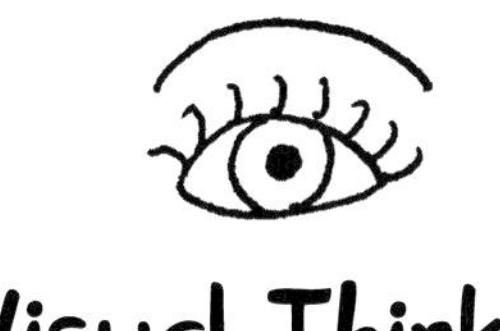

Visual Thinking

I'm a visual thinker. Are you? Author Temple Grandin says visual thinkers see things that allow us to make rapid-fire associations. In short, we think in pictures. This helps with doodling.

Remember a time you relied on pictures, such as driving directions.

Doodle something related to that time.

The Visual Alphabet

After years of research, David Gray invented The Visual Alphabet for doodling. It has 12 shapes, "a common framework for working with more complex ideas." The shapes are below. Duplicate each one.

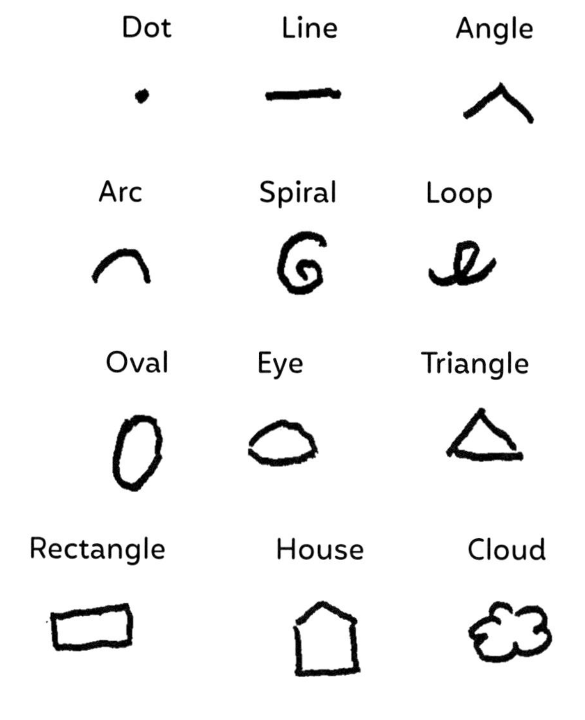

Scribbles, the First Doodles

Close your eyes and scribble here.

The Tight Scribble

Doodle a tight scribble here, as tightly wound as a ball of yarn.

The Loose Scribble

Make a curved scribble here with open spaces. Fill the spaces with doodles.

Calming Lines

Continue the lines until you have filled the page.

Calming Shapes

Choose one of these shapes and fill the page with it. Let your mind wander as you doodle.

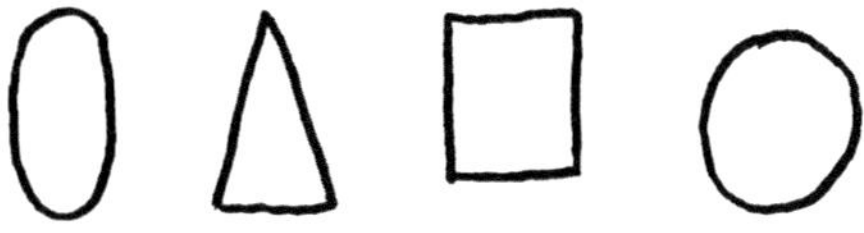

Man in the Moon

Doodle the moon with a face and a cloud or two.

Night of Stars

Doodle different-sized, wonky stars and make them shine.

Kissing Circles

Doodle lots of overlapping circles.
Fill the open spaces with doodle flowers.

Bright Sun

Doodle a second circle around the sun, add rays, and a face.

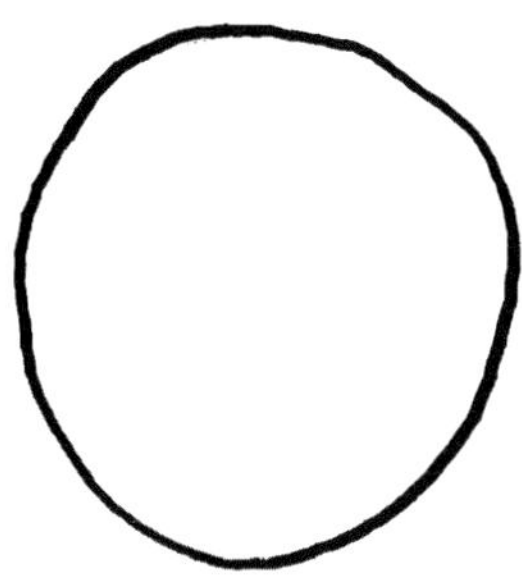

A Dragon Fly Flew By

Dragon flies, an insect with a long body and big, beautiful wings, are beautiful. Doodle one here.

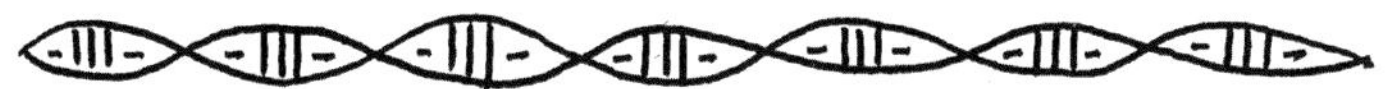

Artful Alphabet Letters

Pick any letter of the alphabet and use it (right-side up, upside down, or sideways) in a doodle. Repeat it often.

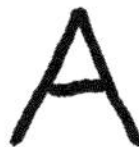

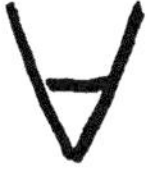

Amazing Oval

One shape, such as an oval, can be riveting. Doodle an oval abstract design or object.

Serene Spirals

Add a different doodle shape
to each spiral.

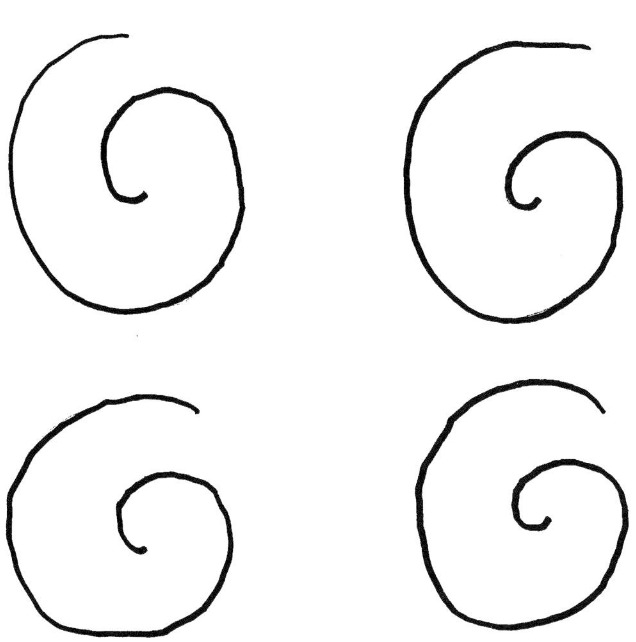

All About Eyes

Doodle two sets of eyes here.

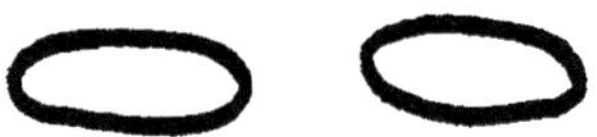

All About Noses

Doodle a different nose on each oval.

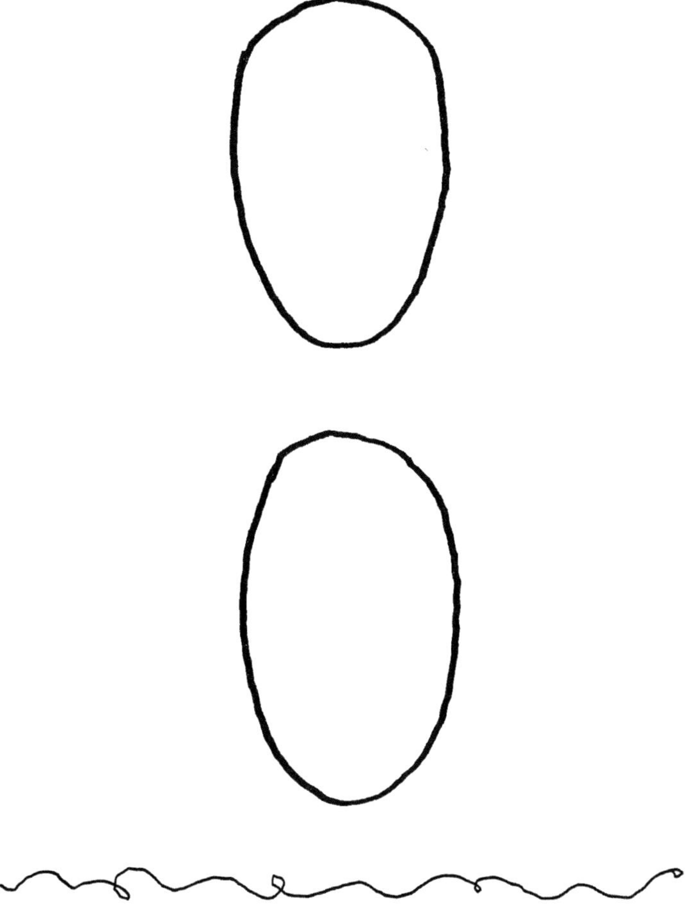

All About Lips

Doodle a different mouth on each oval.

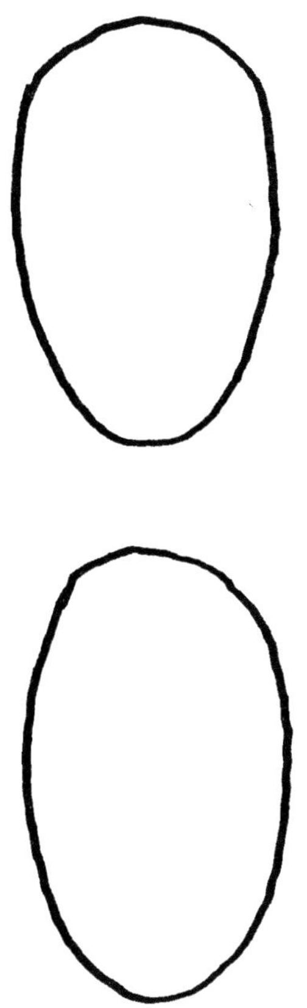

Ms. or Mr. Observant

Doodle big eyes on this face
and other features too.

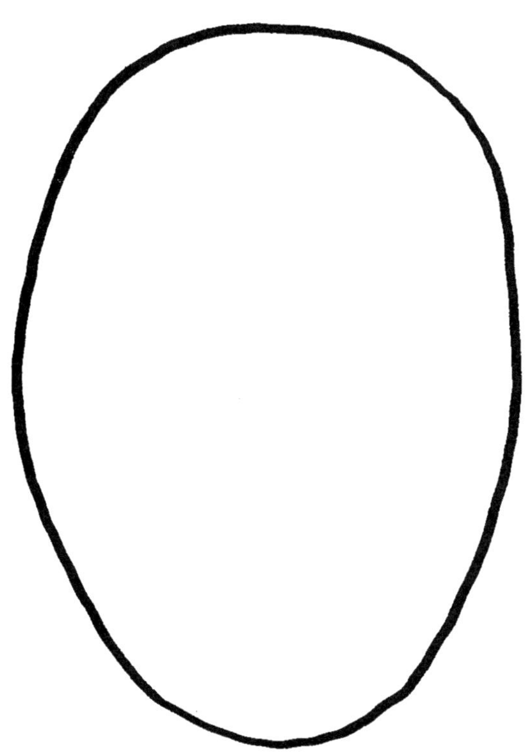

Faces in Spaces

Doodle a scribble with open spaces.
Add a face to each empty space.

Swimming Fish

Turn these geometric shapes into fish by adding doodle lines and patterns.

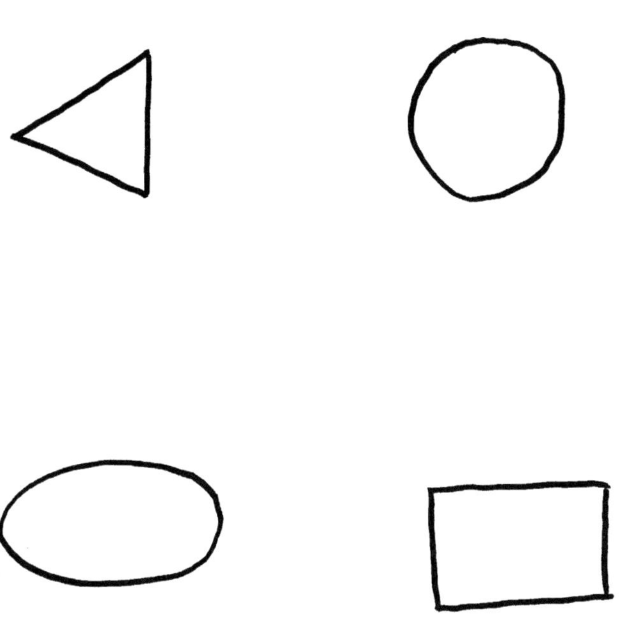

Magical Lines

Lines can be any size, any shape, and anywhere. Fill each square with different doodle lines.

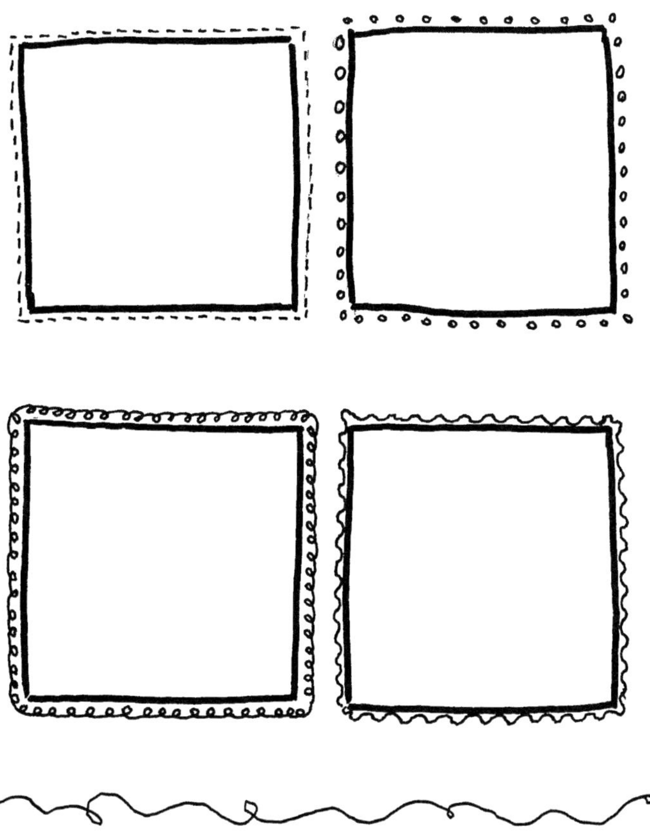

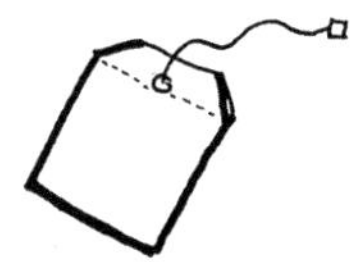

Time for Tea

Doodle a teapot and show the steam rising from the spout with dashes.

Flood Zone!

Doodle water spilling out of this flooded claw-foot bathtub. Doodle the faucet and the water.

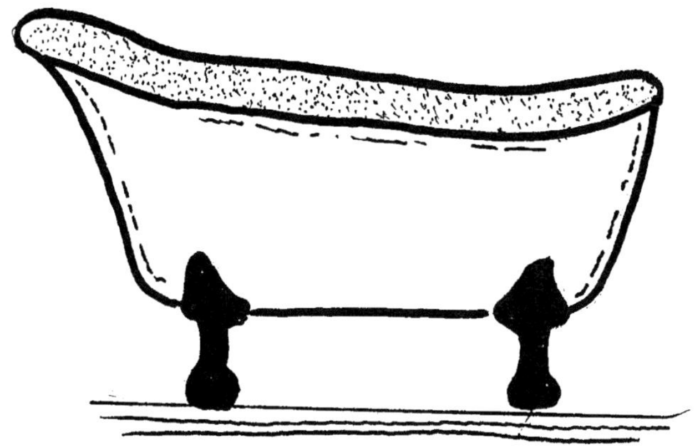

Waves in the Sea

Following the sample, fill this page with waves.

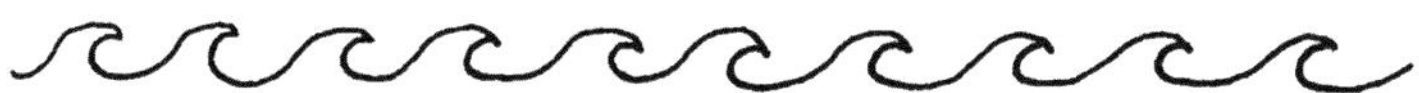

Paisley Birds

Using a variety of doodle techniques, turn these paisley shapes into birds.

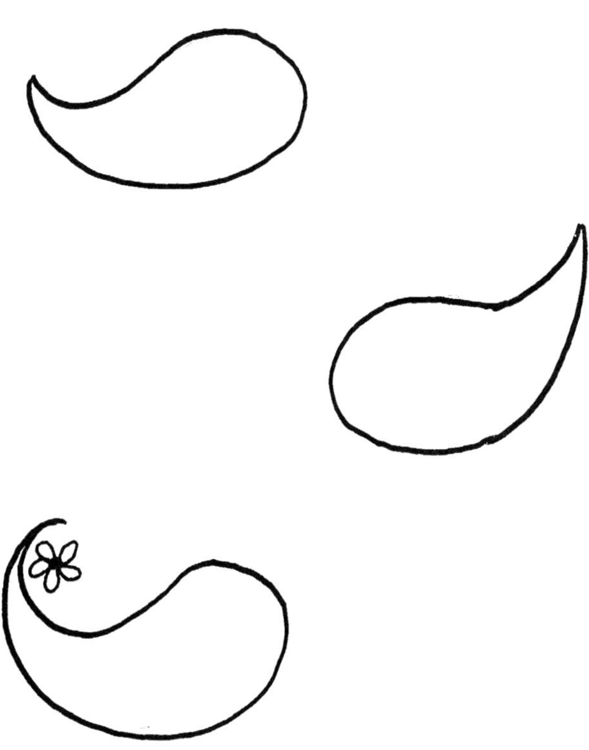

Background Patterns

My favorite backgrounds are circles and asterisks. Practice the background pattern next to each sample.

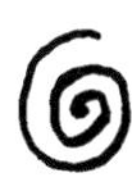

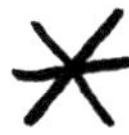

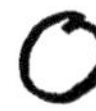

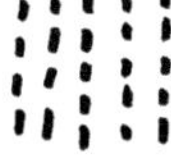

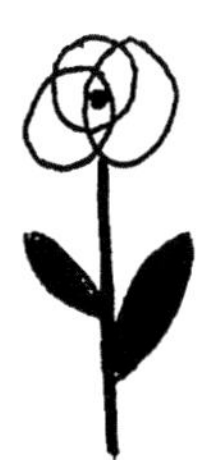

Bud Vase

Doodle a vase with a flower in it and add a background pattern.

Teeny, Tiny Circles

Time to be extra patient. Doodle circular flowers and fill the background with tiny circles.

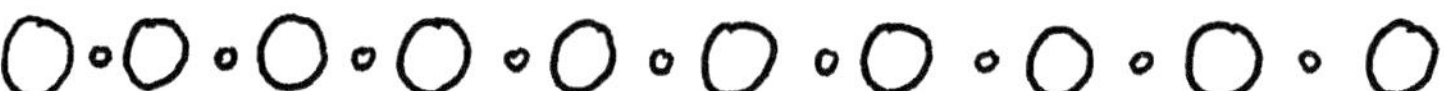

Bland Can Be Beautiful

Find something ordinary and doodle it.

Geometry of Flowers

Study the center of a flower and doodle it.

Focus on The Doodle Alphabet

Choose a shape from The Doodle Alphabet (p.6) and create a doodle that includes this shape. Use it often.

Here's Looking at You

These eyes are a bit scary. What do they belong to? Doodle your answer.

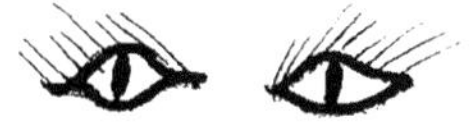

Four-Legged Animal

Doodle a four-legged animal with a tail.

From Your Window

Look out the window and doodle something you see.

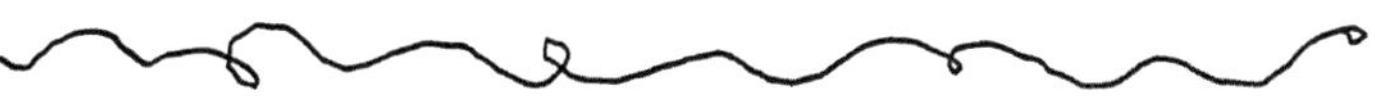

Feathered Friend

Doodle a bird with a swirly, curly tail.

Dots and More Dots

Using dots only, doodle a design here.

Stippling

Doodle more fruit and add tiny dots to show form.

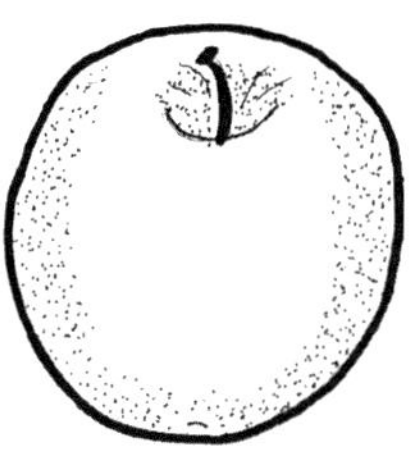

Dot Outlining

Doodle an object and outline it with big dots.

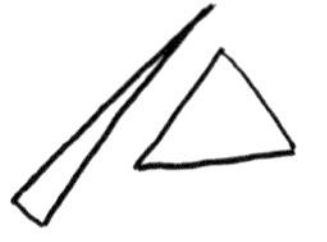

Yikes, it's Spikes!

Doodle a design here with jagged lines and triangles.

Fluffy Clouds

Kids often include cumulous clouds in their drawings. Doodle clouds with hatching lines, as shown below.

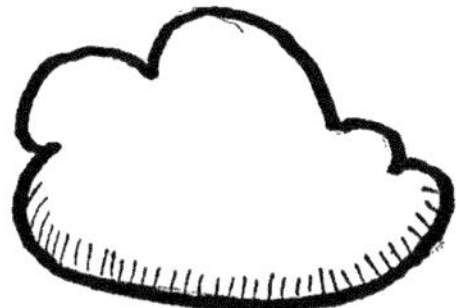

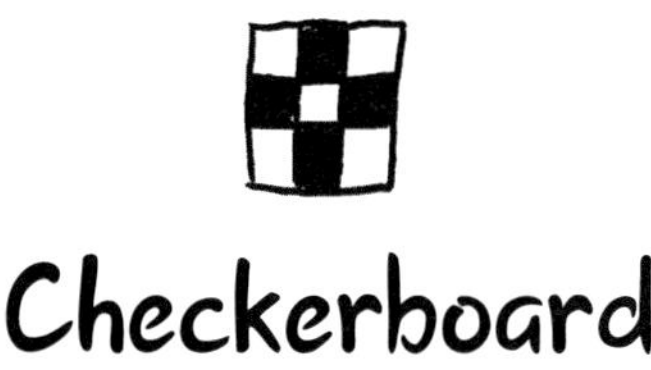

Checkerboard

Create an abstract drawing and include black and white checkerboard squares somewhere.

Spider Web

Doodle inside each wobbly square of this spider web. If you want to, add the spider.

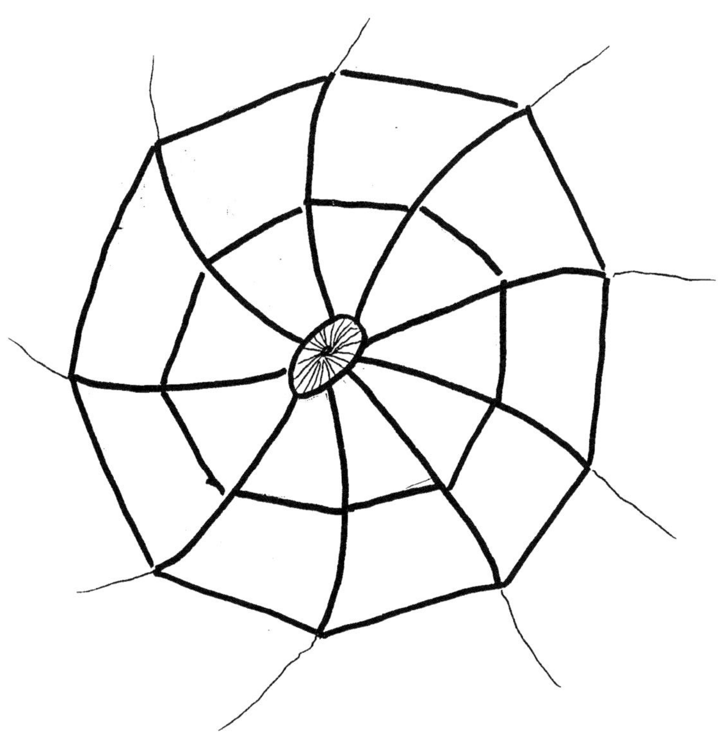

Loop de Loop

Doodle another abstract drawing with loopy lines.

Calming Loops

Continue this loop pattern until you've filled the page.

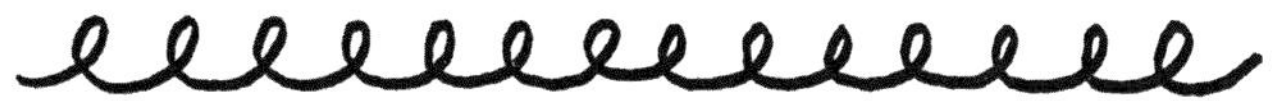

Spirals are Fun

Doodle different sized circles with spirals in the middle.

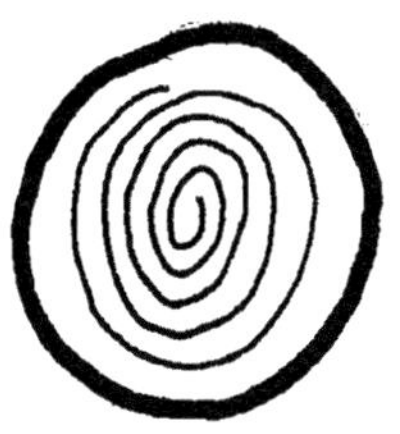

Busy, Buzzing Bee

Doodle dashes to show the flight pattern of this bee. Add another bee.

Heart Mandala

Finish this mandala by adding more circles, flowers, and hearts around the rim.

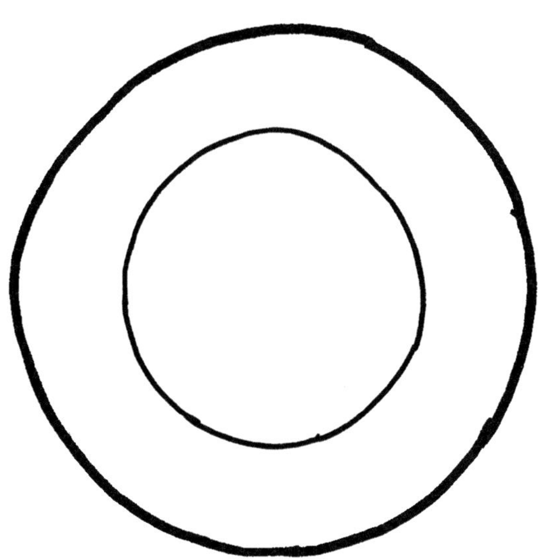

Visual Alphabet Practice

Think of a shape from The Visual Alphabet and doodle it from memory.

Burping Cereal

Doodle loops and shapes to fill this bowl with cereal and decorate the bowl.

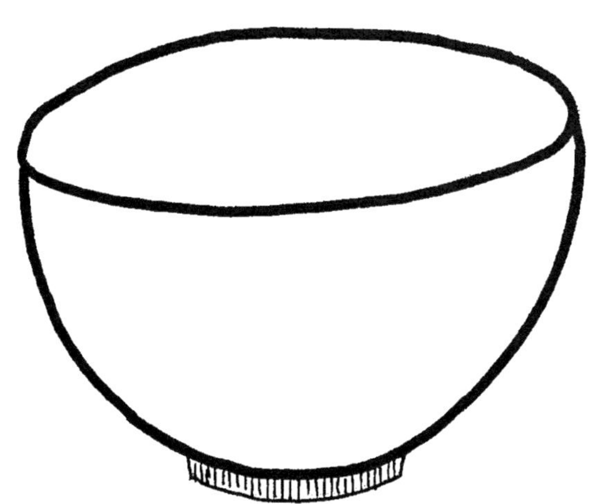

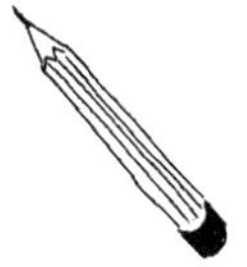

Continuous Line

Keeping your pencil or pen on the paper, make a continuous line doodle. Your doodle may be abstract or recognizable.

Heart's Content

Doodle a different heart design in every square.

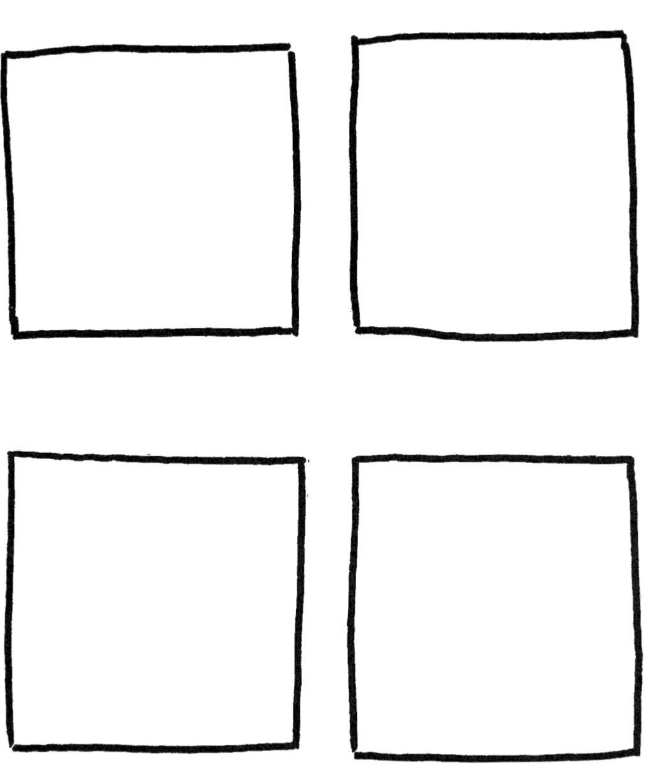

While You're Waiting

Glance at some faces, check the features, and doodle a face.

Growing Creativity

You know trees grow from acorns.
Doodle an oak leaf.

Beautiful Butterfly

Doodle a butterfly and decorate its wings with dots, circles, and lines.

It's Your House

Make this house shape yours by adding doodle details.

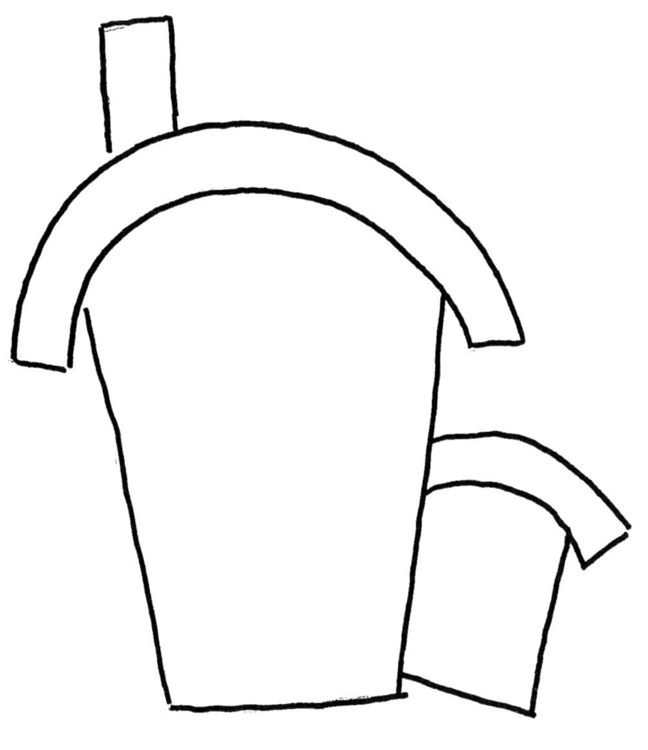

Circles as Borders

Add a circle-dash border to this fame and doodle inside.

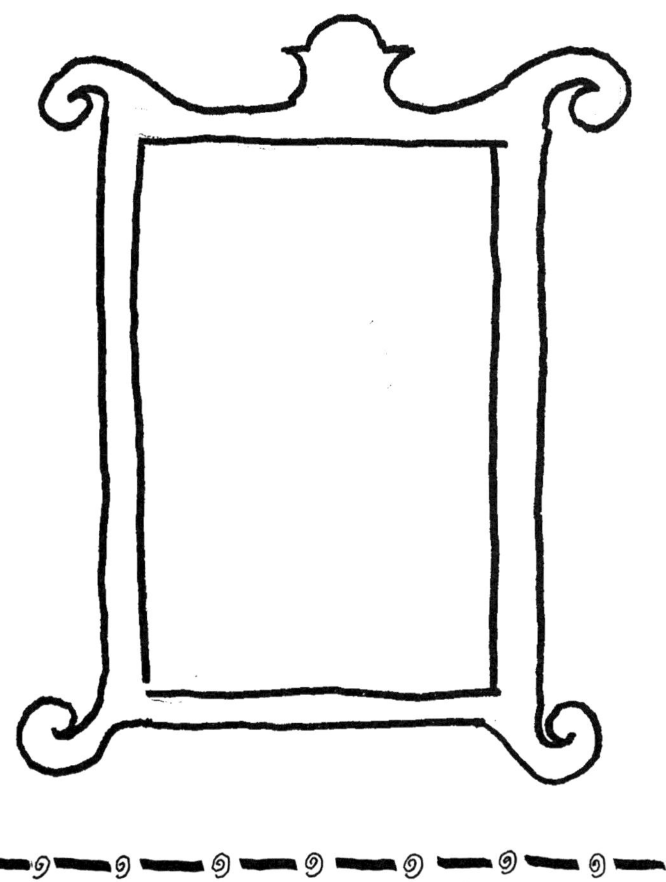

Frame in a Frame

Add doodles to the outside of this frame—right-side up and upside down triangles, curls and dots—whatever you want.

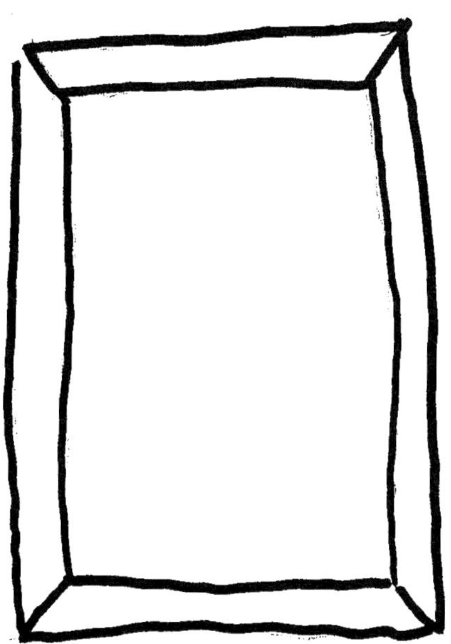

Rainbow After the Storm

Make rainbow lines and fill them with doodles.

Welcome Wreath

Add doodle leaves around this circle to make a wreath.

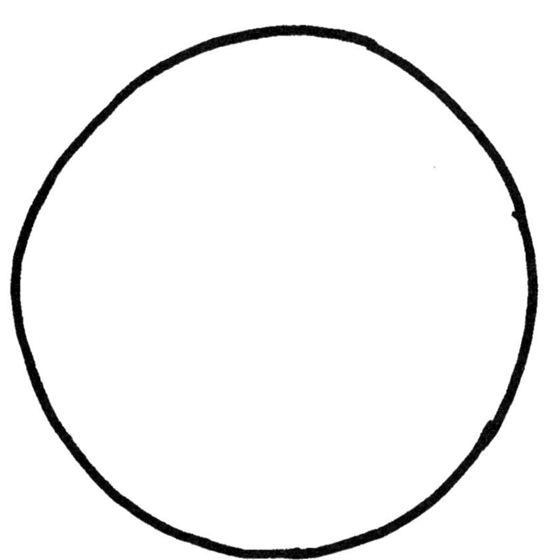

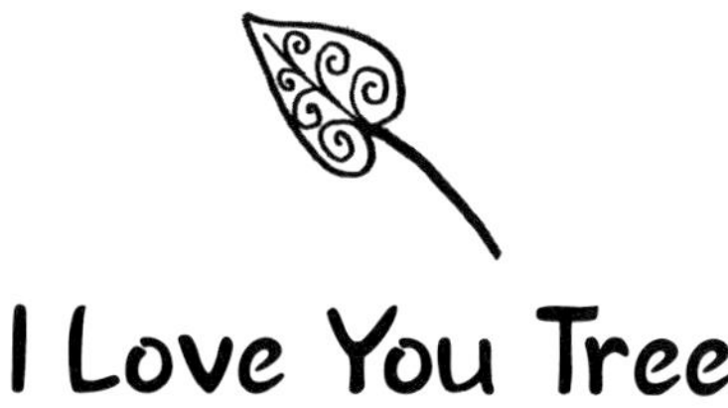

I Love You Tree

Doodle a tree with heart-shaped leaves.

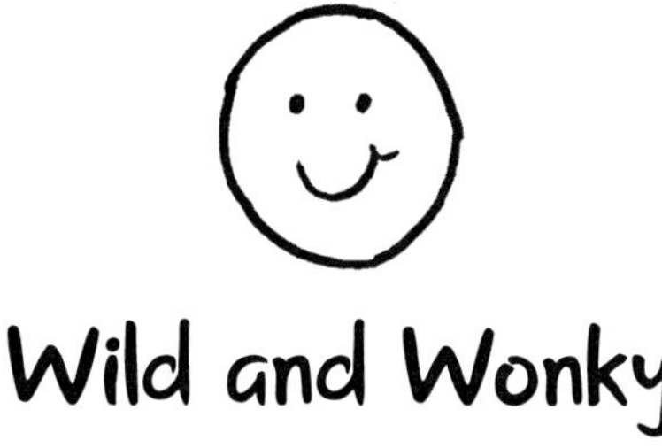

Wild and Wonky

Step out of your comfort zone and surprise yourself with a doodle. It's okay to be wild and wonky with doodles.

Brick by Brick

Finish this brick doodle.

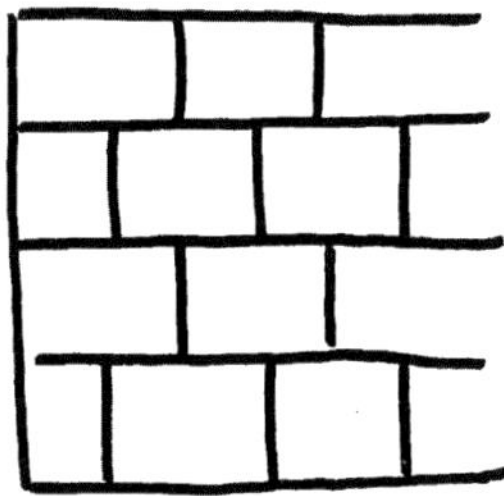

Modern Art

Doodle different kinds of triangles to make a modern art picture.

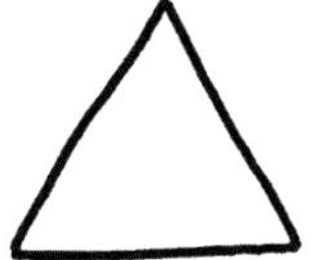

Hidden Alphabet

Create a doodle with hidden alphabet letters as part of the design.

Dancing Arches

Fill the paper with large/small arches and feel the rhythm as you make them.

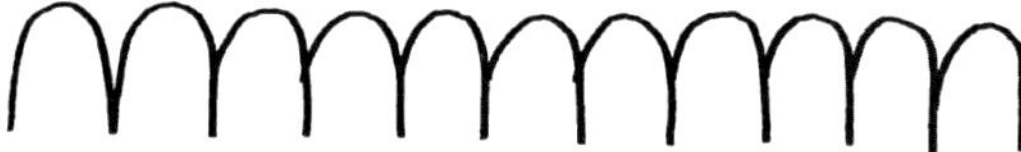

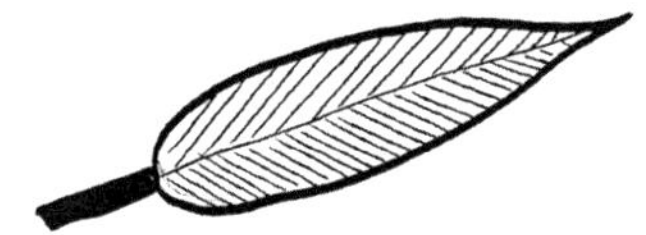

Sweet, Spiral Flowers

Doodle different size spirals and add stems and leaves.

Designer Jeans

Turn these plain jeans into designer jeans by adding doodle shapes and patterns.

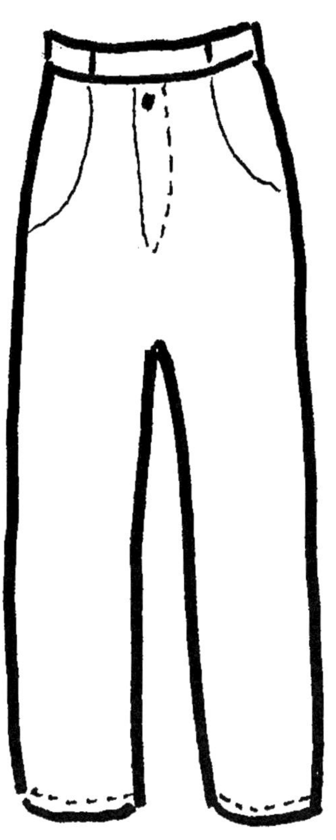

Giant Sunflower

Finish this giant sunflower with doodles.

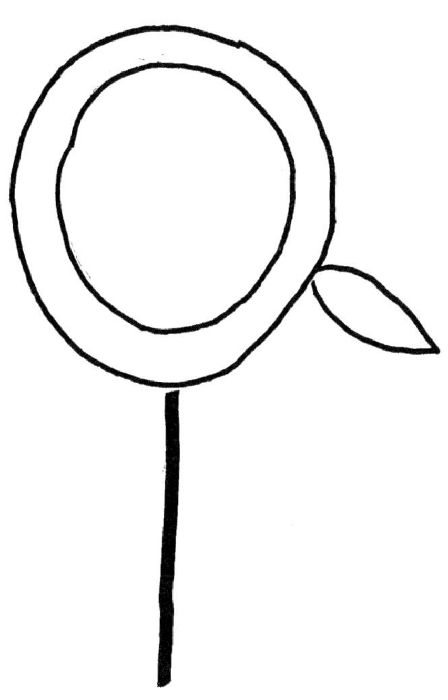

At the Beach

Doodle some waves. Add bubbles and a shell or starfish.

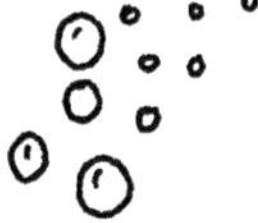

Crazy Quilt

Doodle inside each square of this quilt.
Make some squares "crazy looking."

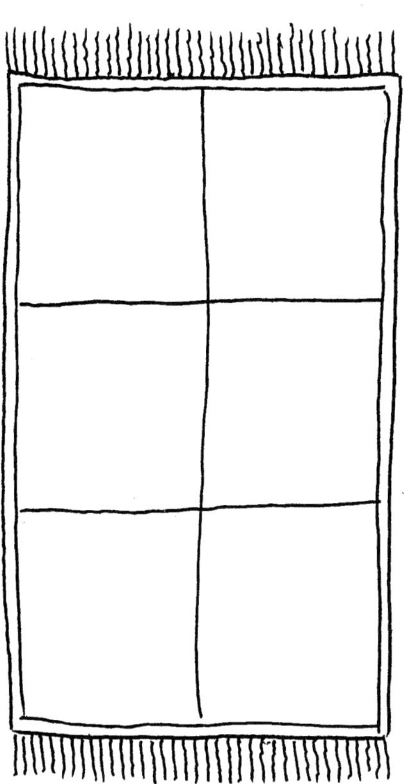

Put on a Happy Face

Doodle a happy male or female face here.

Chubby Birds

Finish and fill these bird silhouettes with doodles.

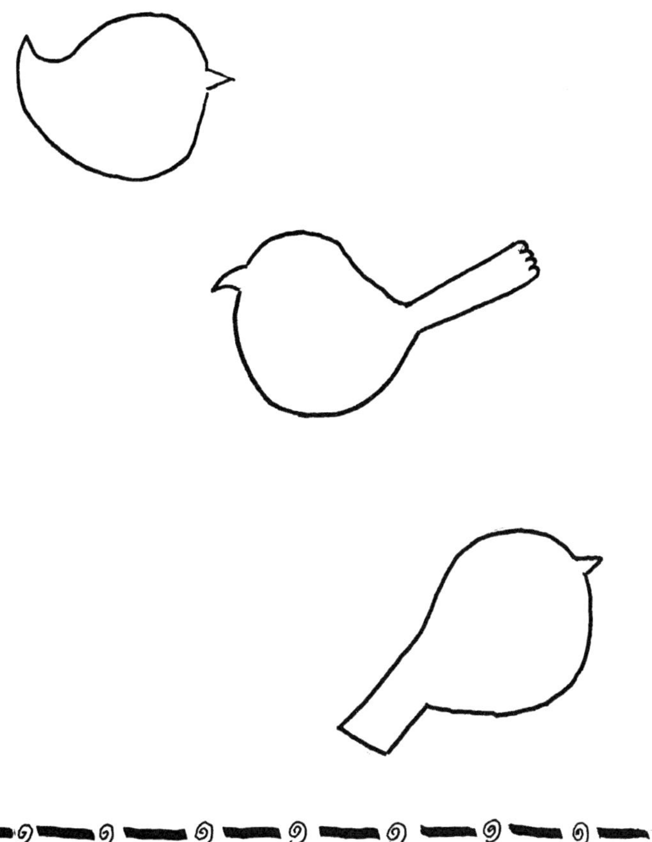

Doodles Tell a Story

Tell a two-part story with doodles.
This (your first doodle) . . .

did this (your second doodle).

Some Sketching Goals

- Continue to practice doodling techniques/patterns.
- Ignore wonky lines and "mistakes."
- Doodle regularly.
- Doodle to calm yourself.
- Try cartoonish doodles, abstract doodles, and folk-art doodles.
- Create larger doodles on larger paper.
- Add interest with colored pencils, markers, watercolors, or watercolor pens.
- Select a favorite doodle and frame it.
- Hang your doodle art where you see it daily.

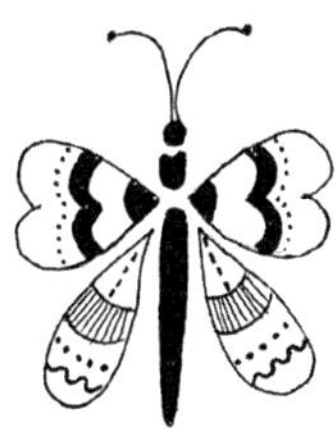

Be Proud of Yourself

These are realistic goals. Be proud of yourself if you keep some or all of them. When you doodle, you're not wasting time, you're saving time.

Doodle yourself here.

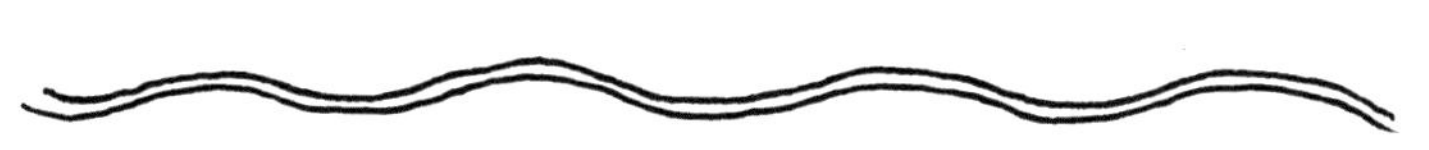

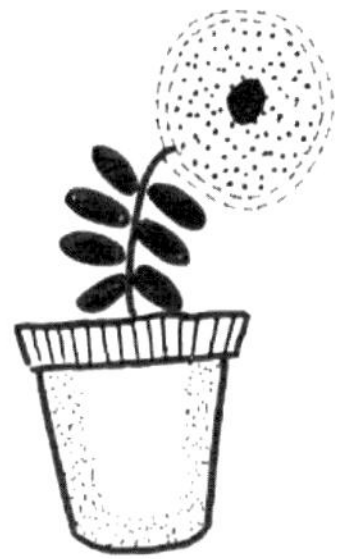

There is no more powerful way to prove that we know something well than to draw a simple picture of it.

— Dan Roam

It took me a lifetime to learn how to paint like a child.

— Pablo Picasso

Resources

Brown, Sunni. *The Doodle Revolution.* New York, Penguin Group, 2015.

Cloud Appreciation Society website, https://cloudappreciationsociety.org

Fink, Joann. *Zenspirations.* Mount Joy, PA. Design Originals, an imprint of Fox Chapel Publishing, 2011.

Grandin, Temple. *Visual Thinking*, New York, Riverhead Books, an imprint of Penguin Random House, 2022.

Gray, David, "In Defense of the Visual Alphabet," https://medium.com/@davegray/in-defense-of-the-visual-alphabet-a8dcca7cf151

Lloyd, Melissa. *Doodle Breaks*, www.doodlebreaks.com, no city or date.

Magsamen, Susan and Ross, Ivy. *Your Brain on Art*. New York, Random House, 2023.

Pillay, Srini, "The 'Thinking' Benefits of Doodling," Harvard Health, Dec. 15, 2016.

Roam, Dan. *On the Back of the Napkin.* New York, Portfolio, 2013.

Scobie, Lorna. *365 Days of Feel-Good Art.* London, Hardie Grant, 2022.

Sokol, Dawn DeVries. *Doodle Zen*. New York, Abrams, 2016.

Vinther, Bianca. "Creativity in Art: The Ultimate Overview," The Pointless Artist website, https://www.thepointlessartist.com/post/creativity-in-art-the-ultimate-overview

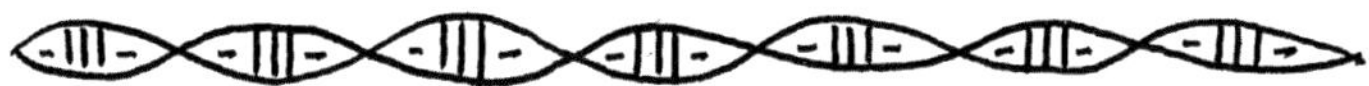

About the Author

Harriet Hodgson is the author of 49 books. She has a BS in Early Childhood Education from Wheelock College of Education and Human Development, MA in Art Education from the University of Minnesota, is an art therapy coach, and busy doodle artist. Visit www.harriethodgson.net for more info.

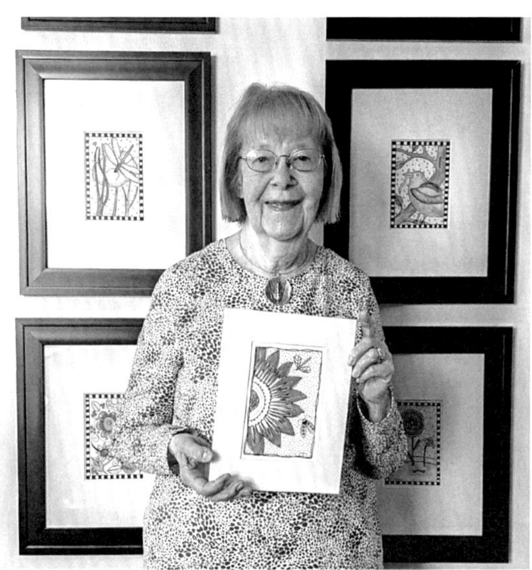